HOW TO REDUCE BELLY FAT FOR MEN: Simple Ways to reduce Belly Fat for men, Based on Science

Rodrigo Monaldo

TABLE OF CONTENT

CHAPTER ONE

AVOID SUGARAND SUGAR-SWEETENED DRINKS

Should We Avoid Sugar to Keep it From Killing Us?
Let me add some perspective:

If you just take studies about the dangers of sugar at face value, sugar does, indeed, look dangerous. Excess sugar consumption is associated with an increased risk of obesity, diabetes, and heart disease. However, when you look a little closer, you find that most of these studies have been done by looking at the correlation of each of these conditions with sugar-sweetened beverage consumption (sodas and fruit juices) (sodas and fruit juices).

A few studies have looked at the correlation between obesity and disease with total "added sugar" consumption. However, 71.6% of added sugar in the American diet comes from sugar-sweetened beverages and junk food. None of the researchers have looked at the sugar in nutritious foods such as fruits, vegetables, and whole grains. That's because there is substantial evidence that these foods lessen the risk of obesity, diabetes, and heart disease.

For example, if apples had a nutrition label, it would list 16 grams of sugar in a medium 80-calorie apple, which corresponds to about 80% of the calories in that apple.

The sugar in an apple is about the same proportion of fructose and glucose found in high fructose corn syrup. Apples are not special. The nutrition label would read roughly the same on most other fruits. Does it imply you should avoid sugar from all fruits? I think not.

Avoid Sugar or Avoid Certain Foods

avoid sugar from junk foodsThe obvious question is: "Why are the same sugars, in nearly the same quantities, harmful in sodas and healthy in fruits?

" Let's go back to those studies I just mentioned—the ones that are often used to vilify sugars.

They are all association studies, on the relationship of sugar consumption with obesity and numerous illnesses.

The weakness of association studies is the association could be with something else that is tightly correlated with the variable (sugar intake) that you are measuring. Could it be the food that is the issue, not the sugar?

If we look at healthy foods (fruits, vegetables, whole grains) they are chock full of vitamins, minerals, phytonutrients, fiber, and (sometimes) protein. Fiber and protein slow the absorption of sugar into the bloodstream.

As a result, blood sugar levels rise slowly and are sustained at relatively low levels for a substantial period.

In sodas, there is nothing to slow the absorption of blood sugar. You get a rapid rise in blood sugar followed by an equally rapid fall. The same is true of junk foods consisting primarily of sugar, refined flour, and/or fat. Avoid sugar from those types of foods.

Another consideration is something called caloric density. Here is a simple analogy.
I used to explain the concept of caloric density to medical students in my teaching days. There are about the same number of calories in a 2-ounce candy bar and a pound of apples (around 278 in the 2-ounce candy bar

and 237 in a pound of apples) (around 278 in the 2-ounce candy bar and 237 in a pound of apples). You can eat a 2-ounce candy bar and still be hungry. If you eat a pound of apples you are done for a while. In this example, the 2-ounce candy bar had a high caloric density (a lot of calories in a tiny container) (a lot of calories in a small package). Perhaps a more familiar terminology would be the candy bar was just empty calories.

Are Sodas and Junk Foods Killing Us? avoid sugar from candyPutting all that together, you may start to realize why the foods the sugars are in are more essential than the sugars themselves. When you consume sugars in the form of sugar-sweetened beverages or sugary junk foods, your appetite increases. We don't know for sure whether it is the intense sweetness of those foods, the rapid increase, and fall in blood sugar, or the high caloric density (lots of calories in a small package) that makes us hungrier.

It doesn't matter. We crave more food, and it isn't usually fruits, vegetables, and complex carbohydrates we crave. It's more trash. That puts in motion a predictable chain of events.

We overeat. Those additional calories are deposited as fat and we become obese. [Note: The low-carb fanatics will tell you that our fat reserves originate from carbs alone. That is wrong. All excess calories, whether from protein, fat, or carbohydrate, are stored as fat.]

It's not simply the fat you can see (belly fat) that is the issue.

Some of that fat builds up in our liver and muscles. This sets up an undesirable cascade of metabolic reactions.

The fat stores release inflammatory cytokines into our bloodstream.

That promotes inflammation. Inflammation increases the risk of many diseases including heart disease and cancer.

The fat deposits also lead our cells to grow resistant to insulin. That lowers the ability of our cells to take in glucose, which leads to hyperglycemia and types 2 diabetes. [Note: The low-carb fanatics will tell you carbs cause type 2 diabetes. That is also inaccurate. It is our fat deposits that induce insulin resistance and type 2 diabetes.

Our fat stores come from all excess calories, not just excess calories from carbohydrates.]

Insulin resistance also causes the liver to overproduce cholesterol and triglycerides and pump them into circulation. That increases the risk of heart disease.

Sugar-sweetened drinks and sugary junk meals also replace healthy items from our diet. That leads to possible nutrient deficiencies that may raise our risk of various illnesses.

However, none of this has to happen. The one thing that every effective diet has in common is the avoidance of beverages, junk foods, quick meals, and convenience foods. You should avoid sugar from such foods as much as possible. Once you eliminate those from your diet, you significantly enhance your chances of being at a healthy weight and being healthy long term.

What About Protein Supplements And Similar Foods?

Of course, the question is what you, as an inquisitive label reader, should do about protein supplements, meal replacement bars, or snack bars. They are supposed to be healthy, but the label lists one or more sugars.

Even worse, the sugar level is greater than your favorite health expert suggests. So, should you avoid sugar from vitamins and the like?

In this scenario, a more relevant idea is the glycemic index, which is a measure of the influence of the meal on your blood sugar levels.

Healthy foods like apples may have high sugar content, but they have a low glycemic index.

Avoid sweets and take protein to limit absorption.
The same is true for the protein pills and bars you are contemplating. Rather than looking at the sugar amount, you should be searching for the words "low glycemic" on the label. That suggests there is enough fiber and protein in the diet to decrease the absorption of sugar into circulation and regulate your blood sugar levels.

What Does This Mean For You?

Don't misinterpret me. I am not advocating for limitless use of sugar. We should focus on strategies to avoid sugar or minimize the quantity of sugar in our diet. On the other hand, we don't need to become so rigorous that we and our families need to consume things that taste like cardboard.

We also don't want to substitute natural sugars with artificial sweeteners. I have warned about the hazards of artificial sweeteners earlier.

We can go a long way towards lowering sugar by merely removing sodas, other sugar-sweetened drinks, junk meals, fast foods, convenience foods, and pastries from our diet. When evaluating quick meals and convenience foods, we should examine the label for hidden sugar. For example, some Starbucks drinks are mostly sugar.

When contemplating foods that are meant to be healthy, we should check for the word "low glycemic" on the label.

So we don't have to eliminate sugar, but we should minimize sugar from sugar-sweetened drinks and junk food.

We need to put warnings about the hazards of sugar in perspective:

The research indicating that sugar intake contributes to obesity, diabetes, and heart disease has all been done using drinks and junk foods.

Many fruits contain just as much sugar as Coke. They also contain nearly the same amount of fructose and glucose as high fructose corn syrup. Yet we know fruits are good for us.

Diets rich in fruits, vegetables, and whole grains minimize our risk of obesity, diabetes, and heart disease.

That is because the sugar in healthy meals is typically present together with fiber and protein, which delays the absorption of sugar and reduces the blood sugar spikes we experience with sodas and junk foods.

In the case of prepackaged meals like protein supplements, you should search for "low glycemic" on the label rather than sugar content. Low glycemic indicates that there is enough fiber and protein in the food to decrease the absorption of sugar and avoid blood sugar increases.

Don't misinterpret me. I am not advocating for limitless use of sugar. We should all focus on strategies to avoid sugar from junk foods or minimize the quantity of sugar in our diet. On the other hand, we don't need to become so rigorous that we and our families need to consume things that taste like cardboard. We also don't want to substitute natural sugars with artificial sweeteners.

We can go a long way towards lowering sugar by merely removing sodas, other sugar-sweetened drinks, junk meals, fast foods, convenience foods, and pastries from our diet. When evaluating quick meals and convenience foods, we should examine the label for hidden sugar. When contemplating foods that are meant to be healthy, we should check for the word "low glycemic" on the label.

CHAPTER TWO

EAT MORE PROTEIN

High protein consumption has various possible health advantages and might assist promote weight reduction, stimulating muscle building, and improving your overall health.

Here are simple methods to consume extra protein.

Eat your protein first

When eating a meal, consume the protein source first, particularly before you get to the carbs.

Protein promotes the synthesis of peptide YY (PYY), a gut hormone that makes you feel full and content.

In addition, a high protein consumption reduces levels of ghrelin, the "hunger hormone," and raises your metabolic rate after eating and throughout sleep.

What's more, eating protein first may help prevent your blood sugar and insulin levels from climbing too high after a meal.

In one tiny trial, patients with type 2 diabetes were offered similar meals on various days. Blood sugar and insulin climbed much less when they ingested protein and vegetables before consuming high-carb items, compared with when the sequence was reversed.

Snack on cheese

Snacks are a fantastic way to incorporate extra protein into your diet – as long as you select healthy ones.

Many typical snack items, such as chips, pretzels, and crackers, are quite low in protein.

For example, a 1-cup (30-gram) meal of plain tortilla chips offers 142 calories but just 2 grams of protein.
In comparison, a 1-ounce (28-gram) portion of cheddar cheese has 7 grams of protein, along with approximately 30 fewer calories and 6 times as much calcium.

Additionally, cheese doesn't appear to boost cholesterol levels significantly, even among persons with high cholesterol. Some studies show that cheese may even enhance heart health

Try savoring a cheese stick between meals or mix your favorite kind of cheese with whole grain crackers, tomatoes, or sliced apples for a nutritious and enjoyable snack.

Replace cereal with eggs
Many morning meals are low in protein, including bread, bagels, and cereals.

Although oatmeal has more protein than other cereals, it still supplies around 5 grams in a normal 1-cup (240-gram) portion.

On the other hand, 3 big eggs give 19 grams of high-quality protein, along with vital minerals like selenium and choline.

What's more, multiple studies have shown that eating eggs for breakfast suppresses hunger and keeps you full for several hours, so you wind up consuming fewer calories later in the day.

According to one earlier research, eating whole eggs might also affect the size and structure of your LDL (bad) cholesterol particles in a manner that may even lessen your heart disease risk.

Top your meals with sliced almonds

Almonds are highly nutritious.

They're strong in magnesium, fiber, and heart-healthy monounsaturated fat, while low in digestible carbohydrates.

Almonds also include 6 grams of protein in a 1-ounce (28-gram) portion, which makes them a superior source of protein to other nuts.

And while a serving of almonds has roughly 170 calories, studies have shown that your body absorbs only around 133 of those calories because part of the fat isn't metabolized.

So sprinkle a few tablespoons of chopped almonds over yogurt, cottage cheese, salads, or oatmeal to enhance your protein intake and add a little taste and crunch.

Choose Greek yogurt
Greek yogurt is a flexible, high-protein snack.

It's prepared by eliminating whey and other liquids to make a richer, creamier yogurt that's higher in protein.

A 7-ounce (240-gram) serving delivers 17–20 grams of protein, depending on the exact brand. This is nearly double the quantity in conventional yogurt.

Research reveals Greek yogurt promotes the production of the gut hormones glucagon-like peptide 1 (GLP-1) and PYY, which suppress appetite and make you feel full.

In addition, it includes conjugated linoleic acid (CLA), which has been demonstrated to enhance the fat reduction in several studies.

Greek yogurt has a tart taste that mixes well with berries or chopped fruit. It may also be used as a replacement for sour cream in dips, sauces, and other dishes.

Have a protein smoothie for breakfast

Many smoothies include a lot of fruit, veggies, or juice, but relatively little protein.

However, a shake or smoothie may be a terrific breakfast alternative, particularly if you pick nutritional components.

Protein powders make it simple to produce a nutritious, high-protein drink. There are various varieties on the market, including whey, soy, egg, and pea protein.

Whey protein powder has been examined the most and appears to have an advantage over the others when it comes to helping you feel full.

In reality, one scoop (28 grams) of whey powder offers roughly 17 grams of protein, on average.

Here's a simple whey shake recipe:

Whey Protein Shake

8 ounces (225 grams) of unsweetened almond milk
1 scoop (28 grams) of whey powder
1 cup (150 grams) of fresh berries
stevia or another healthy sweetener, if desired\s1/2 cup (70 grams) of crushed ice
Combine all ingredients in a blender and process until smooth.

To boost the protein content even further, use extra protein powder or add peanut butter, almond butter, flaxseeds, or chia seeds.

Include a high protein dish with every meal

When it comes to protein, it's not simply the overall quantity you consume every day that counts. Getting enough at each meal is also vital.

Several researchers advocate having a minimum of 20–30 grams of protein at each meal.

Studies suggest that this quantity increases satiety and retains muscle mass better than lesser quantities consumed throughout the day.

Examples of foods strong in protein include meat, fish, poultry, eggs, lentils, and soy products like tofu or tempeh.

You may also choose meals from this list of excellent high-protein foods to make sure you satisfy your requirements at every meal.

Choose leaner, somewhat bigger pieces of meat

Selecting leaner types of meat and raising portion sizes slightly may considerably enhance the protein composition of your meal.

What's more, your meal may even wind up being fewer calories.

For example, compare the nutritional content of a 3-ounce (85-gram) portion of these two steaks:

T-bone steak: 21 grams of protein and 250 calories
Sirloin steak: 26 grams of protein and 150 calories

Add peanut butter to your diet

Peanut butter is a tasty, high-protein snack with a creamy texture that works nicely with a range of toppings.

Studies reveal that peanut butter may be connected with various health advantages and might lower hunger, enhance fat burning, and reduce blood sugar levels.

Peanut butter may also increase the taste and nutritional value of hard fruits like apples and pears, which are rich in fiber and antioxidants but low in protein.

Adding 2 tablespoons (32 grams) of peanut butter over sliced fruit may enhance the total protein amount by 7 grams.

Peanut butter also works well with a broad variety of other items, like oats, celery, whole wheat bread, or yogurt.

Eat lean jerky
Lean jerky is a simple and handy method to incorporate extra protein into your diet.

However, it's crucial to pick a healthy type.

Many forms of jerky include sugar, preservatives, and other problematic components. They're also typically produced from inferior-grade beef.

Some jerky and snack sticks are from grass-fed cattle, bison, and other free-range animals. Choosing jerky from grass-fed animals will deliver superior quality meat with larger quantities of beneficial omega-3 fats.

Lean jerkies or snack sticks offer roughly 9 grams of protein per ounce (28 grams).

They can typically be kept for many months without refrigeration and are extremely portable and suitable for travel.

Indulge in cottage cheese at any moment

Cottage cheese is a delightful dish that's also quite strong in protein. A 1-cup (210-gram) serving includes 23 grams of protein and 176 calories.

A 2015 research revealed cottage cheese to be as full and gratifying as eggs.

What's more, full-fat types are a rich source of CLA, which may assist in fat reduction and contribute to healthier body composition.

One earlier research examined women who ate a high protein, high dairy diet while exercising and lowering calorie consumption. They shed more abdominal fat and built more muscle mass than women with modest amounts of protein and dairy.

Cottage cheese is excellent on its own. You may also try it with chopped nuts or seeds, cinnamon, and stevia for a quick and simple breakfast.

Additionally, smaller portions of cottage cheese make a fantastic snack between meals and may be added to fruit salads or smoothies to ramp up their protein counts.

Munch on edamame

Edamame is the name for steamed soybeans in their unripened condition.

Soybeans provide more protein than other legumes and are popular among vegetarians and vegans.

One cup (155 grams) of edamame offers about 19 grams of protein and roughly 188 calories.

Edamame is also strong in an antioxidant known as kaempferol. Mouse studies show it may lower blood sugar and promote weight reduction.

Edamame may be obtained fresh or frozen and makes an excellent snack. It may also be added to stir-fries, salads, stews, and rice recipes.

Eat canned fish

Canned salmon is a terrific method to enhance your protein consumption.

It needs no refrigeration, so it's ideal for travel. It may also be consumed as a snack or with a meal.

A 3.5-ounce (100-gram) serving of canned salmon has roughly 19 grams of protein and only 90 calories.

Fatty fish like salmon, sardines, herring, and mackerel are also good providers of omega-3 fatty acids, which help combat inflammation and promote heart health.

Ideas for serving canned fish include mixing it with healthy mayo, presenting it on top of a salad, eating it straight from the can, or adding it to an omelet, croquette, or pasta meal.

Enjoy more whole grains
Whole grains are rich in critical nutrients, including fiber, vitamins, minerals, and antioxidants.

What's more, they might also help ramp up your consumption of protein.

For instance, a 1-cup (185-gram) meal of cooked quinoa has 8 grams of protein, but cooked amaranth gives almost 9 grams of protein per cup (246 grams).

This is much higher than refined grains like white rice, which has only 4 grams of protein per cooked cup (158 grams).

Other examples of protein-rich whole grains are buckwheat, couscous, wild rice, millet, and teff.

Try putting these items in for refined grains in dishes like pilafs, stir-fries, and grain salads.

CHAPTER THREE
EAT FEWER CARBOHYDRATES

Here are ways you can cut down on carbohydrates without sacrificing, well, anything:

Cut down on oatmeal amounts by adding flavorful vegetables.
Who says your A.M. do oats have to be sweet? "I almost exclusively eat savory oatmeal,"

"It's full with veggies, [so you can have] half the oats. I use whatever's in season—a couple of days ago I prepared asparagus-dill oatmeal. Use water or vegetable broth instead of milk, and then instead of adding fruit, add veggies. It's like a risotto, but it's a lot simpler to make! You chop the veggies up so you can add it to the water when you add the oats, which take approximately five minutes to cook."

When it comes to a great bagel, concentrate on consuming the right portion amount.

Bagels tend to blast over standard serving proportions, notes Michelle Dudash, R.D., Cordon Bleu-certified chef and founder of Clean Eating Cooking School: Monthly Meal Plans Made Simple. "Have half a bagel, or 'carve' it—pull off the center if you prefer the crust. Cottage cheese is a wonderful topping for bagels, or unsweetened nut butter like peanut butter, almond butter, cashew butter, or walnut butter. Put your fresh fruit on top instead of jelly—lower its in carbohydrates," she advises.

Make yellow squash hash browns.

"Instead of potatoes, you can use yellow summer squash and add anything you would typically add to hash browns," explains Newgent. "I may add green pepper and onion. It looks precisely like a hash brown, but you have fewer carbohydrates [than you do with potatoes]."

Try two-ingredient flour-free pancakes.

Bring on the pancake breakfast. "I've created two-ingredient pancakes with one medium banana, two eggs, and I generally add a sprinkle of salt," adds Newgent. Even though bananas carry carbohydrates, "It's going to be less [than conventional pancakes]. I like to prepare a chocolate version, too, where I add a little cocoa powder. I sprinkle them with honey at the end." Yum!

You may also try this recipe below that adds a cherry and yogurt topping to the morning meal.

Switch up your sandwich bread...
Instead of ordinary bread, go for what many companies term sandwich things. "Whole-wheat or whole-grain sandwich things are wonderful because you get a top and a bottom, and they're low in calories and carbs compared to a typical white bread," explains Koplin. Adds Dudash, "It's handling the portion management for you and they are all approximately 100 calories".

...Or eat your sandwich open-faced.

This may be the oldest technique in the carb-cutting book, but today, it's really sort of nice. "Sometimes instead of a traditional sandwich, an open-faced sandwich is trendier, like a toast or a tartine," explains Newgent. It's also extra pretty—hello avocado toast Instagrams! You may try one of this blog's innovative avocado toast upgrades—get the recipe here.

Portobello mushroom caps may stand in as burger buns.

"What I've done instead of hamburger buns is grilled portobello mushroom caps," explains Newgent. While some people use portobellos in place of patties, you may enjoy your genuine meat, too, with this change. "It looks and functions like a bun, but you want to use a fork and knife," she says.

Order the burrito bowl instead of the entire burrito.

"At a Mexican restaurant, I advocate getting the bowl instead of the burrito, because you're getting the same tastes, but if you're getting beans, rice, and a tortilla, you're getting carbohydrates on carbs on carbs," adds Dudash. Another option? Skip the rice and go for lettuce instead for a delicious salad. And you may try this recipe below, too.

DIY your salad dressing.

Speaking of salad, bottled dressings are typically tricky regarding sugar levels (sugar is a carb) (sugar is a carb). To prevent this, create your vinaigrette for your lunch salad. "My favorite thing to do is blend balsamic vinegar, apple cider vinegar, or red wine vinegar with Dijon mustard, maybe a little bit of honey or agave, and then a sprinkle of olive oil," adds Dudash. "That's my formula for most salad dressings."

Use vegetables as dippers instead of chips.

Instead of using chips or pita for your favorite dip, switch them out and use vegetables instead. Next time you go for hummus, guacamole, or salsa, "you can use romaine hearts, celery, sliced cucumbers, or bell pepper strips—cut them extremely broad so they're like planks," adds Dudash. Making homemade hummus enables you to get creative with the taste, like this miso variation below.

Swap ordinary popcorn with cauliflower popcorn.

Popcorn may be a healthy option when it's air-popped and not filled with butter, salt, and oil, but if you're looking to limit carbohydrates, this swap can provide your the same crispy enjoyment. "I've created cauliflower popcorn," adds Newgent. "You chop cauliflower into little bite-sized pieces and simply bake it until it's crispy, and you can use that in place of popcorn. Top it with olive oil, salt, and a small bit of turmeric, since that'll turn it a little yellow. It has some richness because of the olive oil—it's an adult version of popcorn.

I roast it at 475 degrees for up to 20 minutes until it's golden brown."

Bulk up your spaghetti by mixing it with vegetables.
"Cut down on the spaghetti quantity and [toss it with] cooked veggies," suggests Koplin. "Also put in your lean protein, such as chicken, turkey, or lean ground beef along with your roasted veggies. That's a pretty fantastic approach to bulk up the portion without bulking up the carbohydrates." And top with your favorite sauce (Kroplin enjoys a tomato and basil or garden vegetable red sauce) (Kroplin likes a tomato and basil or garden vegetable red sauce.) Newgent adds, "I'll slice bell peppers extremely thin and put them in the water at the same time as the pasta, so

you're practically boiling them and it becomes part of the process. It tastes a little bit sweeter but then you can sort of balance it with a little additional spice, like red pepper flakes."

You may skip the noodles completely with spiralized veggies...

Spiralized veggies may be used in practically any pasta recipe as a replacement for noodles. "I do very much what I would do with my spaghetti noodles—I just put my veggies and marinara sauce on top, plus some lean mince meat." Try one of these unique spiralized recipes—zucchini, beets, sweet potatoes, and turnips all work nicely.

Use spaghetti squash as a stand-in for pasta.

Spaghetti squash is a simple substitution for spaghetti, but it might be scary to attempt to cut through. Koplin offers a straightforward, no-fuss trick for roasting the veggie: "I cover the entire thing in aluminum foil, place it on a pan with additional aluminum foil, and drop it in the oven at around 400 to 415 degrees. Sometimes it takes 45 minutes to an hour to fully cook, but you can sort of forget about it." When you can pierce the skin with a fork, it's cooked through—and a lot simpler to slice in half. "Start scooping it out with your spoon and cover it with tomato sauce, and you've got a delicious supper," adds Koplin.

If you're searching for a recipe, this zesty pesto is the ideal topping for the thick, savory foundation.

You can prepare low-carb lasagna using zucchini or eggplant.

"You can prep extremely long strips of zucchini or eggplant and use them in lasagna, so for each layer, you can put a layer of thinly sliced veggies," explains Newgent. "You could have two layers of noodles and then two layers of veggies, so it's not an all-or-nothing approach."

Mix heaps of shredded vegetables into your rice or couscous.

Newgent calls this vivid exchange 'confetti couscous.' "

Mix grated, non-starchy veggies in with a typical starchier grain, like rice or couscous, so you cut the carbohydrates but you still have that grain. With couscous, add the grated veggies immediately after you mix the couscous into the water since it doesn't take long to cook (approximately five minutes) (about five minutes). With rice, toss them in towards the end of the cooking process, around five minutes before you're done, or stir them in after you're finished making the rice and put the lid on and let it aside for at least five minutes."

She goes for a multicolored mix with shredded zucchini, yellow summer squash, and carrot.

Or change it out for cauliflower rice.

"I love to cook cauliflower rice," adds Newgent. "You essentially simply pulse raw cauliflower in a food processor until it's a rice consistency or even a couscous consistency, and then sauté it in a pan. It contains a lot fewer carbohydrates [than ordinary rice]. There's no constraint, and you can season it or add herbs according to whatever you're combining it with." Top the cauliflower with anything you'd typically combine with rice—the recipe below asks for curry veggies.

Cut down on potatoes by mixing in other roasted vegetables.

One-pan dinners aren't simply easy—they're a chance to cut less on carb-heavy starches and mix in delectable roasted vegetables. "

One of my favorite [ways to cook a] one-pan supper is to take one entire sweet potato, peel it and slice it into bits, and then put in zucchini squash, carrots, and onion.

I sprinkle it on a skillet, [add olive oil], and season it a little bit. I roast it at 400 degrees for approximately 15 to 20 minutes, then I add chopped turkey kielbasa sausage and cook for about 10 more minutes." You may also mix your protein with whichever veggies you have available.

And use nuts for "breaded" chicken.

"When you bread items like fish or chicken, you can cut down on the carbohydrates by using chopped almonds or almond meal instead of flour," explains Dudash. "It's delicious and crispy and it has a nutty flavor. You can simply cut nuts up extremely tiny or ground them in your food processor, and then sprinkle them with a little oil, spices, and herbs. Then, dip your protein in a whisked egg [and then in the nuts]. Cook at a higher temperature, approximately 450 degrees in a convection oven—for chicken nuggets, I'll do 10 minutes."

And no matter what you're eating, alter your plate order.
This simple mental approach may limit how many carbohydrates you're consuming without even trying.
"Normally, it's customary to go for the carbohydrates first," adds Koplin. "Start by heaping half of your plate

with vegetables and fruit, then dish out your lean protein, and let your carbohydrate be the final portion you place on your plate. By the time you get to that area, there's not a whole lot of spaces.

CHAPTER FOUR

EAT FIBER-RICH FOOD

The Academy of Nutrition and Dietetics recommended taking around 14 grams of fiber for every 1,000 calories you consume daily. This translates to roughly 24 grams of fiber for women and 38 grams for men.

Unfortunately, an estimated 95% of American adults and children don't attain the recommended daily fiber intake. In America, the average daily fiber intake is reported to be 16.2 grams.

What is fiber?
Fiber is a generic word that applies to any form of carbohydrate that your body can't handle.

The fact your body doesn't use fiber for fuel doesn't make it less advantageous to your overall health.

Dietary fiber may deliver the following benefits when you take it:

- Reducing cholesterol. Fiber's existence in the digestive tract may aid lower the body's cholesterol absorption. This is especially true if you take statins, which are medications that lower cholesterol and ingest fiber supplements like psyllium fiber.
- Promoting a healthy weight. High-fiber foods like fruits and vegetables tend to be lower in calories. Also, fiber's presence helps block digestion in the

stomach to help you feel fuller for longer.

- Adding bulk to the digestive system. Those who fight constipation or a generally sluggish digestive system may opt to increase fiber in their diet. Fiber naturally contributes weight to the digestive system, as your body doesn't digest it. This stimulates the intestines.
- Promoting blood sugar control. It could take your body longer to break down high-fiber foods. This helps you maintain more consistent blood sugar levels, which is especially helpful for those with diabetes.
- Reducing gastrointestinal cancer risk. Eating adequate fiber may have preventive effects against

several cancer types, including colon cancer. There are numerous explanations for this, including that some kinds of fiber, such as the pectin in apples, may have antioxidant-like characteristics.

Fiber provides various health benefits, but it's crucial to digest fiber-containing meals gradually for a few days to reduce unpleasant symptoms, such as bloating and gas.

Drinking plenty of water when you boost your fiber intake may also help keep these symptoms at bay.

Here are high-fiber dishes that are both beneficial and pleasant.

Pears (3.1 grams).

The pear is a popular fruit that's both tasty and wholesome. It's one of the top fruit suppliers of fiber.

Fiber content: 5.5 grams in a medium-sized, raw pear, or 3.1 grams per 100 grams.

Strawberries (2 grams)

Strawberries are a pleasant, wholesome option that may be consumed fresh.

Interestingly, they're also among the most nutrient-dense fruits you can ingest, with lots of vitamin C, manganese, and several strong antioxidants. Try some in this banana strawberry smoothie.

Fiber content: 3 grams in 1 cup of fresh strawberries, or 2 grams per 100 grams.

Avocado (6.7 grams)

The avocado is a unique fruit. Instead of being heavy in carbs, it's filled with beneficial fats.

Avocados are exceptionally rich in vitamin C, potassium, magnesium, vitamin E, and various B vitamins. They also provide various health benefits. Try them in one of these fantastic avocado recipes.

Fiber content: 10 grams in 1 cup of raw avocado, or 6.7 grams per 100 grams.

Apples (2.4 grams)

Apples are among the tastiest and most pleasant fruits you can taste. They are also quite rich in fiber.

We especially appreciate them in salads.

Fiber content: 4.4 grams in a medium-sized, raw apple, or 2.4 grams per 100 grams.

Raspberries (6.5 grams)

Raspberries are highly nutritious with a very strong flavor. They're loaded with vitamin C and manganese.

Try putting some into this raspberry tarragon dressing.

Fiber content: One cup of raw raspberries offers 8 grams of fiber or 6.5 grams per 100 grams.

Bananas (2.6 grams)

Bananas are a rich source of various nutrients, including vitamin C, vitamin B6, and potassium.

A green or unripe banana also carries a considerable amount of resistant starch, a sort of indigestible carbohydrate that behaves like fiber. Try them in a nut butter sandwich for a punch of protein, too.

Fiber content: 3.1 grams in a medium-sized banana, or 2.6 grams per 100 grams.

Other high-fiber fruits

Blueberries: 2.4 grams per 100-gram serving

Blackberries: 5.3 grams per 100-gram serving.

Carrots (2.8 grams)

The carrot is a root vegetable that's tasty, crisp, and highly healthful.

It's high in vitamin K, vitamin B6, magnesium, and beta carotene, an antioxidant that is turned into vitamin A in your body.

Toss some sliced carrots into your next veggie-loaded soup.

Fiber content: 3.6 grams in 1 cup of raw carrots, or 2.8 grams per 100 grams.

Beets (2.8 grams)

The beet, or beetroot, is a root vegetable that's high in numerous vital elements, such as folate, iron, copper, manganese, and potassium.

Beets are also rich in inorganic nitrates, which are nutrients proven to offer diverse benefits linked to blood pressure control and exercise performance.

Give them a go in this lemon dijon beet salad.

Fiber content: 3.8 grams per cup of raw beets, or 2.8 grams per 100 grams.

Broccoli (2.6 grams)

Broccoli is a sort of cruciferous vegetable and one of the most nutrient-dense foods in the world.

It's rich in vitamin C, vitamin K, folate, B vitamins, potassium, iron, and manganese and has antioxidants and potent cancer-fighting elements.

Broccoli is also fairly high in protein, compared with other vegetables. We like converting them into slaws for diverse uses.

Fiber content: 2.4 grams per cup, or 2.6 grams per 100 grams.

Artichoke (5.4 grams)

The artichoke doesn't make headlines very regularly. However, this vegetable is plentiful in several nutrients and is one of the world's top suppliers of fiber.

Just wait until you try them roasted.

Fiber content: 6.9 grams in 1 raw globe or French artichoke, or 5.4 grams per 100 grams.

Brussels sprouts (3.8 grams)
The Brussels sprout is a cruciferous vegetable that's connected to broccoli.

They're exceptionally strong in vitamin K, potassium, folate, and potent cancer-fighting antioxidants.

Try out Brussels sprouts roasted with apples and bacon or dusted with balsamic vinegar.

Fiber content: 3.3 grams per cup of raw Brussels sprouts, or 3.7 grams per 100 grams.

Other high-fiber vegetables
Almost all vegetables have large quantities of fiber. Other significant cases include:

Kale: 3.6 grams
Spinach: 2.2 grams
Tomatoes: 1.2 grams.
All values are given for raw vegetables.

Lentils (7.3 grams)
Lentils are very affordable and among the most nutritious meals.

They're especially rich in protein and loaded with numerous vital nutrients.

This lentil soup is spiced up with cumin, coriander, turmeric, and cinnamon.

Fiber content: 13.1 grams per cup of cooked lentils, or 7.3 grams per 100 grams.

Kidney beans (6.8 grams)
Kidney beans are a major kind of legume. Like other legumes, they're rich in plant-based protein and other nutrients.

Fiber content: 12.2 grams per cup of cooked beans, or 6.8 per 100 grams.

Split peas (8.3 grams)
Split peas are created from the dried, split, and peeled seeds of peas. They're typically seen in split pea soup after holidays with ham.

Fiber content: 16.3 grams per cup of cooked split peas, or 8.3 per 100 grams.

Chickpeas (7 grams)
Chickpea is another form of legume that's rich in nutrients, including minerals and protein.

Chickpeas are the base of hummus, one of the easiest spreads to create yourself. You may spread it over salads, veggies, whole grain bread, and more.

Fiber content: 12.5 grams per cup of cooked chickpeas, or 7.6 per 100 grams.

Other high-fiber legumes
Most legumes are rich in protein, fiber, and various minerals. When properly prepared, they're among the world's cheapest sources of healthy sustenance.

Other high fiber legumes include:

Cooked black beans: 8.7 grams
Cooked edamame: 5.2 grams
Cooked lima beans: 7 grams
Baked beans: 5.5 grams.

Quinoa (2.8 grams)

Quinoa is a pseudo-cereal that has become quite popular among health-conscious folks in the last several years.

It's rich in various nutrients, including protein, magnesium, iron, zinc, potassium, and antioxidants, to name a few.

Fiber content: 5.2 grams per cup of cooked quinoa, or 2.8 per 100 grams.

Oats (10.1 grams)

Oats are among the healthiest grain foods on the earth. They're incredibly rich in vitamins, minerals, and antioxidants.

They contain a powerful soluble fiber called beta-glucan, which has great beneficial impacts on blood sugar and cholesterol levels.

Overnight oats have become a cornerstone for basic breakfast alternatives.

Fiber content: 16.5 grams per cup of raw oats, or 10.1 grams per 100 grams

Popcorn (14.4 grams)
If your purpose is to enhance your fiber consumption, popcorn may be the finest snack you can have.

Air-popped popcorn is extremely high in fiber, calories for calories. However, if you add a lot of fat, the fiber-to-calorie ratio will decline considerably.

Fiber content: 1.15 grams per cup of air-popped popcorn, or 14.4 grams per 100 grams.

Other high-fiber grains
Nearly all whole grains are high in fiber.

Almonds (13.3 grams)
Almonds are a common kind of tree nut.

They're especially rich in various nutrients, including healthy fats, vitamin E, manganese, and magnesium. Almonds may also be transformed into almond flour for baking with a dosage of extra nutrients.

Fiber content: 4 grams per 3 tablespoons, or 13.3 grams per 100 grams.

Chia seeds (34.4 grams)
Chia seeds are small black seeds that are enormously popular in the natural health movement.

They're highly nutritious, having considerable levels of magnesium, phosphorus, and calcium.

Chia seeds may potentially be the single greatest source of fiber on the globe. Try them paired with jam or some homemade granola bars.

Fiber content: 9.75 grams per ounce of dried chia seeds, or 34.4 grams per 100 grams.

Other high-fiber nuts and seeds
Most nuts and seeds contain high quantities of fiber. Examples include:

Fresh coconut: 9 grams
Pistachios: 10 grams
Walnuts: 6.7 grams
Sunflower seeds: 11.1 grams
Pumpkin seeds: 6.5 grams.
All statistics are for a 100-gram portion.

Sweet potatoes (2.5 grams)
The sweet potato is a popular tuber that's fairly filling and has a fantastic

sweet flavor. It's incredibly rich in beta carotene, B vitamins, and other minerals.

Sweet potatoes may be a great bread substitution or base for nachos.

Fiber content: A medium-sized boiling sweet potato (without skin) yields 3.8 grams of fiber or 2.5 grams per 100 grams.

Dark chocolate (10.9 grams)
Dark chocolate is undoubtedly one of the world's most beautiful desserts.

It's also startlingly high in nutrients and one of the most antioxidant- and nutrient-rich foods on the earth.

Just be sure to choose dark chocolate that has a cocoa content of 70–95% or above and avoid chocolates that are packed with added sugar.

Fiber content: 3.1 grams in a 1-ounce piece of 70–85% cacao, or 10.9 grams per 100 grams.

Fiber is a vital element that may promote weight loss, lower blood sugar levels, and avoid constipation.

Most persons don't attain the recommended daily consumption of 25 grams for women and 38 grams for men.

Try adding any of the aforementioned products to your diet to immediately enhance your fiber intake.

CHAPTER FIVE

EXERCISE REGULARLY

Here are the ways regular exercise improves your body and brain.

Exercise may make you feel happy

Exercise has been proven to enhance your mood and minimize emotions of despair, anxiety, and stress.

It creates changes in the areas of the brain that control stress and anxiety. It may also enhance brain sensitivity to the neurotransmitters serotonin and norepinephrine, which decrease symptoms of despair.

Additionally, exercise may enhance the synthesis of endorphins, which are known to help promote happy moods and lower the perception of pain.

Interestingly, it doesn't matter how tough your exercise is. It appears that exercise may enhance your mood no matter the intensity of the physical activity.

In fact, in research on 24 women diagnosed with depression, the exercise of any intensity dramatically improved symptoms of sadness.

The effects of exercise on mood are so potent that choosing to exercise (or not) even makes a difference over short periods.

One assessment of 19 research indicated that active adults who quit exercising regularly reported substantial increases in symptoms of despair and anxiety, even after just a few weeks.

Exercise may assist with weight reduction

Some studies have indicated that inactivity is a key contributor to weight gain and obesity.

To comprehend the influence of exercise on weight loss, it is vital to understand the link between activity and energy expenditure.

Your body spends energy in three ways:

digesting food

exercising\smaintaining biological functions, such as your pulse, and breathing

While dieting, a decreased calorie intake can lower your metabolic rate, which might temporarily postpone weight reduction. On the contrary, regular exercise has been demonstrated to raise your metabolic rate, which may burn more calories to help you lose weight.

Additionally, studies have shown that combining aerobic exercise with strength training may enhance fat reduction and muscle mass maintenance, which is vital for keeping the weight off and retaining lean muscle composition.

Exercise is healthy for your muscles and bones

Exercise has a critical function in establishing and maintaining healthy muscles and bones.

Activities like weightlifting may boost muscle development when accompanied by proper protein intake.

This is because exercise helps release hormones that enhance your muscles' capacity to absorb amino acids.
This helps them flourish and inhibits their breakdown.

As individuals age, they tend to lose muscle mass and function, which may contribute to an increased risk of injury. Practicing regular physical exercise is vital to decreasing muscle loss and preserving strength as you age.

Exercise also helps improve bone density while you're younger, in addition to helping prevent osteoporosis later in life.

Some studies show that high-impact exercise (such as gymnastics or running) or odd-impact sports (such as soccer and basketball) may assist produce a greater bone density than no-impact sports like swimming and cycling.

Exercise may enhance your energy levels
Exercise may be a great energy enhancer for many individuals,

including those with different medical issues.

One earlier research revealed that 6 weeks of regular exercise improved symptoms of exhaustion for 36 persons who previously experienced continuous fatigue.

And let's not forget the amazing heart and lung health advantages of exercise. Aerobic exercise enhances the cardiovascular system and promotes lung function, which may greatly aid with energy levels.

As you move more, your heart pumps more blood, supplying more oxygen to your working muscles. With frequent exercise, your heart gets more effective and competent at transporting oxygen into your blood, making your muscles more efficient.

Over time, this aerobic training results in reduced stress on your lungs, and it needs less energy to execute the same tasks – one of the reasons you're less likely to feel short of breath during strenuous exercise.

Additionally, exercise has been demonstrated to enhance energy levels in persons with various diseases, such as cancer.

Exercise may minimize your chances of chronic illness

Lack of regular physical exercise is a key cause of chronic illness.

Regular exercise has been demonstrated to enhance insulin sensitivity, heart health, and body composition. It may help lower blood pressure and cholesterol levels.

More precisely, exercise may help lessen or avoid the following chronic health issues.

- Type 2 diabetes. Regular aerobic exercise may postpone or prevent type 2 diabetes. It also provides great health advantages for those with type 1 diabetes. Resistance training for type 2 diabetes involves improvements in fat mass, blood pressure, lean body mass, insulin resistance, and glycemic control.

- Heart illness. Exercise decreases cardiovascular risk factors and is also a therapeutic therapy for persons with cardiovascular disease.
- Many forms of cancer. Exercise may help lower the risk of numerous cancers, including breast, colorectal, endometrial, gallbladder, kidney, lung, liver, ovarian, pancreatic, prostate, thyroid, gastric, and esophageal cancer.
- High cholesterol. Regular moderate-intensity physical exercise may enhance HDL (good) cholesterol while

preserving or balancing increases in LDL (bad) cholesterol. Research supports the hypothesis that high-intensity aerobic exercise is required to reduce LDL levels.

- Hypertension: Participating in regular aerobic exercise may reduce resting systolic BP by 5–7 mmHG among patients with hypertension.
- In contrast, a lack of regular exercise — even in the short term — may lead to considerable increases in belly fat, which may raise the risk of type 2 diabetes and heart disease.

That's why regular physical exercise is suggested to reduce abdominal fat and lessen the chance of getting these diseases.

Exercise may enhance skin health

Your skin might be influenced by the level of oxidative stress in your body.

Oxidative stress arises when the body's antioxidant defenses cannot fully repair the cell damage produced by chemicals known as free radicals. This might harm the structure of the cells and badly influence your skin.

Even though extreme and strenuous physical activity might add to oxidative damage, frequent moderate exercise can improve your body's production of natural antioxidants, which assist protect cells.

In the same manner, exercise may promote blood flow and generate skin cell changes that can help postpone the appearance of skin aging.

Exercise may boost your brain health and memory
Exercise helps increase brain function and preserve memory and cognitive abilities.

To begin with, it boosts your heart rate, which enhances the flow of blood and oxygen to your brain. It may also boost the synthesis of hormones that enhance the proliferation of brain cells.

Plus, the capacity of exercise to avoid chronic illness might translate into advantages for your brain, as its function can be impaired by these disorders.

Regular physical exercise is particularly crucial in older persons as aging — along with oxidative stress and inflammation — causes changes in brain structure and function.

Exercise has been proven to encourage the hippocampus, a portion of the brain that's crucial for memory and learning, to increase in size, which may aid enhance mental performance in older individuals.

Lastly, exercise has been proven to minimize changes in the brain that may lead to illnesses like Alzheimer's disease and dementia.

Exercise may aid with relaxation and sleep quality

Regular exercise might help you relax and sleep better.

Regarding sleep quality, the energy depletion (loss) that happens during exercise drives restorative processes during sleep.

Moreover, the rise in body temperature that happens during exercise is considered to enhance sleep quality by helping body temperature decline during sleep.

Much research on the effects of exercise on sleep has found similar findings.

One evaluation of six research revealed that engaging in an exercise training program helped enhance self-reported sleep quality and lowered sleep latency, which is the amount of time it takes to fall asleep.

One research done over 4 months indicated that both stretching and resistance exercise contributed to improvements in sleep for persons with chronic insomnia.

Getting back to sleep after awakening, sleep length, and sleep quality increased following both stretching and resistance exercises.

Anxiety was also lowered in the stretching group.

CHAPTER SIX

TRACK YOUR FOOD INTAKE

Tracking your food consumption will provide you insight into many areas of your eating habits. The more exact you are with reporting, the more accurate your information will be. You may begin to realize that you are missing whole dietary categories (i.e veggies, dairy) (i.e vegetables, dairy). If you are not sure what is advised, educate yourself on what you need. Each food group provides us with nutrients crucial for maintaining health, so choose nutrient-dense foods from all five food groups.

Do not forget to monitor all the tiny extras; coffee creamer and sugar, condiments, sweets from your coworker's candy stash, drinks, etc. You may be astonished to find out how many calories are in these neglected pleasures. As little as 100 additional calories might translate to 10 extra pounds each year. These are also simple products to cut out or switch with healthier ones.

Tracking food intake will also show you what you are doing well already. Continue with these behaviors so that you don't have to start from scratch. Building on what you are currently doing and taking small steps to improve your eating habits will help you to be more successful!